HEAL YOURSELF
BY YOURSELF

Embracing Wholeness: A Holistic Approach to Wellness, Exploring the interconnectedness of mind, body, and spirit for overall well-being.

FRANCIS WHITE

Copyright © 2024 by Francis White

All rights reserved. No part of this publication may be reproduced, distributed, or transmitted in any form or by any means, including photocopying, recording, or other electronic or mechanical methods, without the prior written permission of the author or publisher, except in the case of brief quotations embodied in critical reviews and certain other noncommercial uses permitted by copyright law.

Disclaimer: The information provided in this book is for educational and informational purposes only. It is not intended to be a substitute for professional medical advice, diagnosis, or treatment. Always seek the advice of your physician or other qualified health provider with any questions you may have regarding a medical condition. Never disregard professional medical advice or delay in seeking it because of something you have read in this book.

TABLE OF CONTENT

INTRODUCTION 6

CHAPTER ONE 9

Understanding Holistic Wellness 9

Defining holistic wellness: 9

Principles of Holistic Wellness: 9

The Interconnectedness of Mind, Body, and Spirit: 12

CHAPTER TWO 16

Nourishing Your Body 16

The Importance of Nutrition in Holistic Wellness: 16

Choosing Whole Foods: 18

Mindful Eating Practices: 20

Exploring Dietary Supplements and Superfoods: 22

3 |Heal yourself by yourself

CHAPTER THREE 26

Cultivating Mental Clarity and Emotional Balance 26

Managing Stress through Mindfulness and Meditation: 26

Techniques for Enhancing Mental Resilience: 29

Strategies for Emotional Self-Care: 32

The Power of Positive Thinking: 35

CHAPTER FOUR 39

Physical Vitality and Movement 39

Finding Joy in Movement: 39

Exploring Different Forms of Physical Activity: 41

The Benefits of Regular Exercise: 44

CHAPTER FIVE 47

Nurturing Relationships and Community 47

The Importance of Social Connections:........47

Building Supportive Relationships: 49

Communication Skills for Healthy Interactions: 51

CHAPTER SIX 54

Environmental Harmony 54

Creating a Healthy Living Environment: 54

Connecting with Nature: 57

Sustainable Living Practices: 59

CHAPTER SEVEN..63

Integrating Holistic Wellness into Daily Life ..63

Practical Tips for Everyday Holistic Living: 63

Overcoming Common Obstacles: 65

CHAPTER EIGHT..72

Beyond the Self: Holistic Wellness for the Greater Good..72

The Ripple Effect of Your Wellness: 72

Advocacy and Activism for a Healthier World: 74

CONCLUSION 78

Embracing Wholeness 78

Reflecting on Your Journey to Holistic Wellness: 78

Committing to Ongoing Growth and Self-Discovery: 79

INTRODUCTION

Welcome to Harmony Within: Cultivating Balance for Mind, Body, and Spirit.

In our fast-paced modern world, it's easy to become disconnected from ourselves and the world around us. We often find ourselves caught in a whirlwind of responsibilities, stressors, and distractions, leaving little time to nurture our well-being. But amidst the chaos, there exists a profound truth: true wellness comes from within.

Heal yourself by yourself is more than just a book; it's a guide to reclaiming your sense of balance, wholeness, and vitality. Drawing upon the principles of holistic living, this book offers a roadmap for integrating mind, body, and spirit in pursuit of optimal health and well-being.

Throughout these pages, you'll embark on a transformative journey of self-discovery and empowerment. You'll learn how to nourish your body with wholesome foods, cultivate mental clarity and emotional resilience, and embrace movement as a pathway to physical vitality. You'll explore the importance of nurturing relationships and fostering connections with your community, as well as creating a harmonious living environment that supports your well-being.

But Harmony Within goes beyond the individual self. It recognizes that our well-being is intimately connected to the well-being of our planet and our communities. As you read through these pages, you'll discover how your journey toward wellness can ripple outwards, creating positive change in the world around you.

Whether you're seeking relief from stress, inspiration for healthy living or guidance on the path to personal growth, Harmony Within offers a wealth of wisdom, practical insights, and transformative practices to support you on your journey.

So, take a deep breath, and let's embark on this journey together. Within these pages, you'll find the tools, resources, and inspiration you need to cultivate harmony, balance, and well-being in every aspect of your life.

CHAPTER ONE

Understanding Holistic Wellness

Defining holistic wellness: Holistic wellness is a comprehensive approach to health and well-being that considers the whole you — body, mind, emotions, and spirit — as interconnected and interdependent. Rather than focusing solely on treating symptoms or addressing specific health concerns in isolation, holistic wellness seeks to promote balance and harmony across all aspects of your life.

At its core, holistic wellness recognizes that optimal health is not merely the absence of disease, but rather a state of dynamic equilibrium in which you experience vitality, resilience, and fulfillment.

Principles of Holistic Wellness: This approach takes into account various factors that contribute to overall well-being; Holistic living is a lifestyle approach that considers the entire you and your overall well-being—physical, mental, emotional, and spiritual—rather than focusing on individual aspects separately.

Physical Health: Holistic wellness encompasses practices and behaviors that support physical health, such as nutritious eating, regular exercise, adequate sleep, and preventive care.

Mental and Emotional Well-being: Mental and emotional health are integral components of holistic wellness. Practices such as mindfulness, stress management, emotional expression, and cognitive reframing are emphasized to promote psychological resilience and balance.

Spiritual Fulfillment: For many individuals, spiritual well-being plays a significant role in their overall sense of wellness. This may involve exploring one's purpose and values, engaging in spiritual practices or rituals, and fostering a sense of connection to something greater than oneself.

Social Connections: Human beings are inherently social creatures, and strong social connections are essential for holistic wellness. Cultivating supportive relationships, fostering a sense of community, and engaging in meaningful social interactions are all vital aspects of this approach.

Environmental Harmony: Holistic wellness extends beyond you to encompass the environment in which you live. This includes creating a healthy living environment, minimizing exposure to toxins and pollutants, and fostering a connection to nature.

Natural Healing Modalities: Holistic living often incorporates alternative and complementary therapies, such as acupuncture, herbal medicine, massage therapy, yoga, meditation, and energy healing. These modalities aim to support your body's innate healing mechanisms and promote balance and harmony.

Quality Relationships: Holistic living values nurturing meaningful connections with oneself, others, and the world around us. Cultivating supportive relationships, fostering empathy and compassion, and practicing effective communication are integral to holistic well-being.

Holistic View of Success: Holistic living encourages a broader definition of success beyond material wealth and external achievements. It emphasizes fulfillment, purpose, and alignment with your values and passions as key indicators of success.

By embracing the principles of holistic living, you can cultivate a lifestyle that supports your holistic well-being and fosters a sense of balance, harmony, and vitality in all areas of life.

The Interconnectedness of Mind, Body, and Spirit:
The interconnectedness of mind, body, and spirit is a fundamental concept in holistic health and wellness. Here's a deeper exploration of each component and how they are interconnected:

Mind: The mind encompasses your thoughts, beliefs, perceptions, emotions, and consciousness. It influences your behaviors, attitudes, and experiences. The mind-body connection highlights that mental states, such as stress, anxiety, or happiness, can impact physical health. For example, chronic stress can weaken the immune system, increase inflammation, and contribute to various health conditions. Practices like mindfulness meditation, cognitive-behavioral therapy, and positive visualization can help harness the power of the mind to promote healing and well-being.

Body: The body refers to the physical aspect of our being, including organs, tissues, cells, and physiological processes. The body-mind connection emphasizes how physical health and well-being are influenced by factors such as nutrition, exercise, sleep, and environmental factors. For instance, regular physical activity not only improves cardiovascular health and strengthens muscles but also enhances mood, reduces stress, and supports cognitive function. Similarly, a balanced diet rich in nutrients fuels the body with essential energy and supports optimal functioning of bodily systems.

Spirit: The spirit encompasses your inner essence, sense of purpose, values, beliefs, and connection to something greater than yourself. It represents the spiritual dimension of human experience, which may manifest as a connection to nature, a higher power, or a deeper sense of meaning and purpose in life.

Spirituality is often associated with qualities like compassion, gratitude, forgiveness, and inner peace.

Cultivating spiritual well-being can contribute to overall health and resilience by providing a sense of meaning, hope, and transcendence in the face of adversity.

The interconnectedness of mind, body, and spirit suggests that these aspects of your experience are not separate entities but are deeply intertwined and mutually influence each other. For example:

Emotional distress (mind) can manifest as physical symptoms such as headaches, muscle tension, or digestive issues (body).

Engaging in physical activities like yoga or tai chi can not only improve physical fitness but also promote relaxation, mindfulness, and emotional balance (mind).

Practices like meditation, prayer, or spending time in nature can foster a sense of inner peace, connectedness, and spiritual fulfillment (spirit).

By recognizing and nurturing the interconnectedness of mind, body, and spirit, you can cultivate holistic well-being and promote health on multiple levels—physically, mentally, emotionally, and spiritually. This integrated approach to health and wellness acknowledges the complexity of your experience and the importance of addressing the whole you in promoting health and healing.

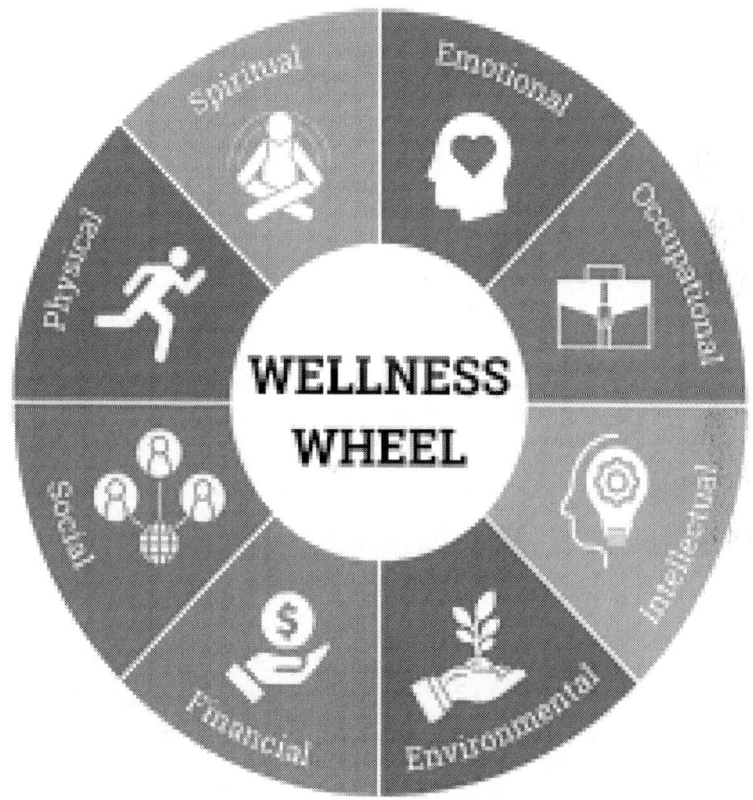

15 |Heal yourself by yourself

CHAPTER TWO

Nourishing Your Body

The Importance of Nutrition in Holistic Wellness: Nutrition plays a crucial role in holistic wellness, as it directly impacts the interconnected aspects of mind, body, and spirit. Reasons why nutrition is essential in holistic wellness:

Physical Health: Nutrition provides your body with essential nutrients, vitamins, minerals, and energy needed for optimal functioning. A balanced diet supports organ health, boosts the immune system, maintains healthy weight, and reduces the risk of chronic diseases such as heart disease, diabetes, and certain cancers.

Mental Clarity and Emotional Balance: The food you eat can influence cognitive function, mood, and emotional well-being. Nutrient-rich foods, such as fruits, vegetables, whole grains, and healthy fats, support brain health and cognitive function, while minimizing processed foods, sugar, and artificial additives can help stabilize mood and reduce the risk of mental health conditions like depression and anxiety. Nutrient-rich foods, particularly those high in omega-3 fatty acids, antioxidants, and vitamins, support brain health, enhance memory, concentration, and mental clarity, and reduce the risk of cognitive decline and neurodegenerative diseases. Conversely, poor nutrition, such as diets high in processed foods, sugar, and unhealthy fats, can impair cognitive function, mood stability, and mental well-being.

Emotional Well-being: Nutrition plays a significant role in regulating mood and emotions. Certain foods contain nutrients that can influence neurotransmitter levels in the brain, such as serotonin and dopamine, which are associated with feelings of happiness and well-being. A balanced diet can help stabilize your mood and reduce the risk of mental health disorders like depression and anxiety.

Energy Levels: The foods we eat directly affect our energy levels. Nutrient-dense foods provide sustained energy throughout the day, while sugary or processed foods can lead to energy crashes. Maintaining stable energy levels through proper nutrition enhances productivity and overall vitality.

In essence, nutrition is the cornerstone of holistic wellness, influencing every aspect of your physical, mental and emotional health. By making informed food choices and prioritizing a balanced diet, you can optimize your well-being and lead fulfilling lives.

Choosing Whole Foods: Whole foods are essential to holistic wellness because, it prioritizes nourishing your body with nutrient-dense, minimally processed foods that support overall health.

Nutrient Density: Whole foods are rich in essential nutrients like vitamins, minerals, antioxidants, and fiber, which are vital for optimal health. These nutrients work synergistically to support various bodily functions and promote overall wellness.

Digestive Health: Whole foods are typically easier to digest than processed foods since they contain natural enzymes, fiber, and other compounds that support digestive health. A healthy digestive system is important for absorption of nutrient and overall well-being.

Blood Sugar Regulation: Whole foods, such as fruits, vegetables, whole grains, and lean proteins, tend to have a lower glycerin index compared to processed foods. This means they cause a slower and steadier rise in blood sugar levels, which is beneficial for managing energy levels and preventing insulin spikes and crashes.

Balanced Nutrition: Whole foods offer a balance of macronutrients (carbohydrates, proteins, and fats) and micronutrients (vitamins and minerals) in their natural form. This balance is required for maintaining energy levels, supporting metabolism, and promoting overall health.

Reduced Exposure to Harmful Ingredients: Processed foods often contain additives, preservatives, artificial colors, and flavors that may have negative effects on your health when consumed in excess. Choosing whole food helps minimize exposure to these potentially harmful substances.

Mind-Body Connection: Holistic wellness considers the interconnectedness of mind, body, and spirit.

Eating whole foods can positively impact mental well-being by providing essential nutrients that supports brain function and mood regulation.

Environmental Sustainability: Whole foods, especially when sourced locally and sustainably, have a lower environmental impact compared to heavily processed and packaged foods. Choosing whole foods supports environmental sustainability by reducing energy consumption, greenhouse gas emissions, and waste production.

Prioritizing whole foods in your diet aligns with the principles of holistic wellness by nourishing your body with natural, nutrient-rich foods that support overall health and well-being, while also considering the broader impact on the environment and the interconnectedness of mind, body, and spirit.

Mindful Eating Practices: Mindful eating is all about being present and fully engaging with the experience of eating. Here are some practices to cultivate mindfulness while eating:

Engage your senses: Pay attention to the appearance, aroma, and sounds of your food. Take a moment to appreciate the appearance and aroma before taking a bite.

Eat slowly: Chew your food thoroughly and savor each bite. Put your utensils down between bites to slow down the pace of your meal.

Focus on the experience: Avoid distractions like TV, Smartphone, or reading while eating. Instead, focus your attention solely on the act of eating and the sensations it brings.

Listen to your body: Play in to your body's hunger and fullness cues. Eat when you're hungry and stop when you're satisfied, rather than eating out of habit or boredom.

Be non-judgmental: Approach your eating experience with curiosity and kindness, without judgment or criticism of yourself or your food choices.

Appreciate where your food comes from: Consider the journey your food took to reach your plate, from the farm to the store to your table. Appreciating this can deepen your connection to your food and increase gratitude.

Practice gratitude: Take a moment before eating to express gratitude for your meal, whether it's for the food itself, the people who prepared it, or the circumstances that allowed you to have it.

Pause midway: Midway through your meal, pause for a moment to check in with yourself. Notice how you're feeling physically and emotionally. Are you still hungry? Are you enjoying the flavors?

Be mindful of portion sizes: Pay attention to portion sizes and how much food you're putting on your plate. Eat only what you need to satisfy your hunger, rather than mindlessly overeating.

Reflect after eating: Take a moment to reflect on your eating experience after you've finished your meal. How do you feel? What did you enjoy most about the meal? Is there anything you would do differently next time?

Incorporating these practices into your daily meals can help you develop a more mindful approach to eating, leading to greater enjoyment, satisfaction, and overall well-being.

Exploring Dietary Supplements and Superfoods: Exploring dietary supplements and superfoods can be an exciting journey toward optimizing your health and well-being.

Dietary Supplements:

Vitamins and Minerals: These are micronutrients essential for various bodily functions. Common examples include vitamin C, vitamin D, iron, calcium, and magnesium. While it's best to obtain nutrients from a balanced diet, supplements can be helpful for filling gaps in your nutrition.

Herbal Supplements: Derived from plants, herbal supplements are used for various purposes, including immune support, stress reduction, and improved digestion. Examples include Echinacea, ginseng, and turmeric.

Omega-3 Fatty Acids: Found in fish oil supplements, omega-3 fatty acids are beneficial for heart health, brain function, and reducing inflammation.

Probiotics: These are live bacteria and yeasts that are good for your digestive system. Probiotic supplements can help restore the natural balance of gut bacteria and improve digestion.

Superfoods:

Berries: Blueberries, strawberries, raspberries, and other berries are packed with antioxidants, vitamins, and fiber, offering numerous health benefits including improved heart health and brain function.

Leafy Greens: Spinach, kale, Swiss chard, and other leafy greens are rich in vitamins, minerals, and phytonutrients, promoting overall health and reducing the risk of chronic diseases.

Nuts and Seeds: Almonds, walnuts, flaxseeds, and hemp seeds are excellent sources of healthy fats, protein, and fiber, supporting heart health and weight management.

Fatty Fish: Salmon, mackerel, and sardines are rich in omega-3 fatty acids, which are essential for brain health, heart health, and reducing inflammation.

Avocado: Avocados are packed with healthy fats, fiber, and vitamins, promoting heart health, weight management, and skin health.

Quinoa: A nutritious whole grain, quinoa is high in protein, fiber, and various vitamins and minerals, making it an excellent addition to a balanced diet.

When exploring dietary supplements and superfoods, it's essential to remember that while they can complement a healthy diet, they're not a substitute for it. Prioritize whole, nutrient-dense foods in your diet, and consult with a healthcare professional before adding supplements, especially if you have underlying health conditions or are taking medications.

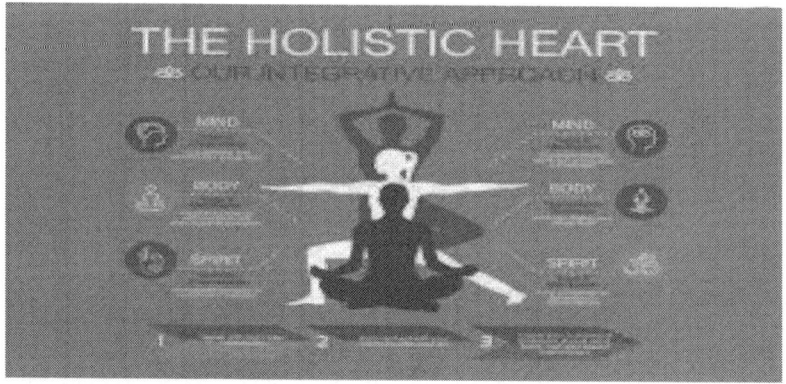

CHAPTER THREE

Cultivating Mental Clarity and Emotional Balance

Managing Stress through Mindfulness and Meditation: Managing stress through mindfulness and meditation can be incredibly beneficial for both mental and physical well-being. How mindfulness and meditation can help, along with some practical tips for incorporating them into your routine:

Awareness of the Present Moment: Mindfulness involves paying attention to the present moment without judgment. By focusing on the here and now, you can reduce the tendency to dwell on past regrets or worry about the future, which are common sources of stress.

Stress Reduction: Meditation practices, such as deep breathing, exercises or body scans, activate the body's relaxation response, which counteracts the stress response. This can lead to reduced levels of stress hormones like cortisol and lower blood pressure.

Improved Emotional Regulation: Mindfulness and meditation can help you develop greater emotional awareness and regulation. Instead of reacting impulsively to stressful situations, you can learn to respond more calmly and thoughtfully.

Enhanced Resilience: Regular mindfulness and meditation practice can build resilience to stress over time. By strengthening your ability to stay present and centered, you become better equipped to handle life's challenges with grace and composure.

Increased Self-Compassion: Mindfulness encourages self-compassion, which involves treating yourself with kindness and understanding, especially during difficult times. This can help counteract negative self-talk and reduce feelings of self-criticism that contribute to stress.

Ways for incorporating mindfulness and meditation into your daily routine:

Begin Small: Start by dedicating a few minutes each day to meditation or mindfulness practice, and progressively extend the length as you feel increasingly at ease.

Choose a Consistent Time: Establish a regular meditation schedule by choosing a time of day that works best for you, whether it's first thing in the morning, during a lunch break, or before bed.

Find a Quiet Space: Create a quiet, comfortable space where you can meditate without distractions. This could be a designated meditation corner in your home or simply a quiet room where you can sit comfortably.

Experiment with Different Techniques: There are many different meditation techniques to probe, including mindfulness meditation, loving-kindness meditation, and body scan meditation. Experiment with different techniques to find what works most with you.

Be Patient and Persistent: Just like any other skill, mindfulness and meditation require practice and patience. Be kind to yourself and don't get discouraged if your mind wanders or if you find it challenging at first.

Simply acknowledge any distractions and gently guide your focus back to the present moment.

By incorporating mindfulness and meditation into your daily routine, you can cultivate greater resilience, emotional well-being, and overall stress reduction.

Techniques for Enhancing Mental Resilience: Enhancing mental resilience is crucial for navigating life's challenges with strength and adaptability. Techniques that can help boost mental resilience:

Cultivate a Growth Mindset: Embrace the belief that challenges are opportunities for growth rather than insurmountable obstacles. Adopting a growth mindset allows you to view setbacks as temporary and solvable, fostering resilience in the face of adversity.

Practice Self-Compassion: Always remember to treat yourself with kindness and understanding, especially during difficult times. Self-compassion involves acknowledging your own struggles without judgment and offering yourself the same care and support you would give to a friend.

Develop Strong Social Connections: Nurture supportive relationships with friends, family, and community members. Social support is a powerful buffer against stress and can provide emotional validation, encouragement, and practical assistance during challenging times.

Cultivate Optimism: Cultivate a positive perspective by directing your attention towards what you have influence over, and uncovering the positives within challenging circumstances. Optimism doesn't mean denying reality; rather, it involves reframing setbacks as temporary and surmountable, leading to greater resilience in the face of adversity.

Build Emotional Awareness and Regulation Skills: Practice mindfulness and emotional regulation techniques to become more aware of your thoughts and feelings and to respond to them in healthy ways. Techniques such as deep breathing, progressive muscle relaxation, and meditation can help calm the mind and body during times of stress.

Set Realistic Goals and Take Action: Break larger goals into smaller, manageable steps and take proactive steps toward achieving them.

By focusing on achievable tasks and making progress, you can build confidence and a sense of control over your circumstances, bolstering resilience.

Maintain Healthy Habits: Prioritize self-care by getting enough sleep, eating a balanced diet, exercising regularly, and engaging in activities that bring you joy and fulfillment. Physical health and mental well-being are closely intertwined, and maintaining healthy habits can help build resilience.

Seek Meaning and Purpose: Reflect on your values, passions, and long-term goals to find meaning and purpose in your life. Connecting with a sense of purpose can provide a source of motivation and resilience during challenging times.

Practice Adaptability and Flexibility: Cultivate the ability to adapt to changing circumstances and embrace uncertainty. Rather than resisting change, approach it with curiosity and openness, recognizing that adaptation is a natural part of life.

Seek Professional Support When Needed: If you're struggling to cope with stress or facing significant challenges, don't hesitate to seek support from a therapist, counselor, or mental health professional. They can provide guidance, validation, and practical strategies for building resilience and coping effectively with adversity.

Strategies for Emotional Self-Care: Emotional self-care is essential for maintaining mental well-being and resilience. Strategies to prioritize emotional self-care:

Identify Your Emotions: Take time to recognize and acknowledge your emotions without judgment. Being aware of what you're feeling can help you address your needs and respond to challenges more effectively.

Practice Self-Compassion: Treat yourself with kindness and understanding, especially during difficult times. Practice self-compassionate self-talk and recognize that it's normal to experience a range of emotions, both positive and negative.

Set Boundaries: Establish healthy boundaries in your relationships and daily life to protect your emotional well-being. Learn to say no to commitments or activities that drain your energy or cause stress, and prioritize activities that replenish you.

Engage in Activities That Bring Joy: Make time for activities that nourish your soul and bring you happiness. Whether it's spending time in nature, pursuing a creative hobby, or connecting with loved ones, prioritizing joy can boost your emotional resilience.

Practice Mindfulness and Meditation: Incorporate mindfulness and meditation into your daily routine to cultivate awareness of the present moment and promote emotional balance. Mindfulness practices can help you stay grounded and centered, even in the midst of stress or chaos.

Express Yourself Creatively: Engage in creative outlets such as writing, drawing, painting, or playing music to express your thoughts and emotions. Creative expression can be therapeutic and provide a healthy outlet for processing difficult feelings.

Connect with Supportive Relationships: Nurture relationships with friends, family, or support groups who provide validation, empathy, and understanding. Sharing your feelings with trusted individuals can help alleviate loneliness and provide emotional support.

Prioritize Self-Care Activities: Make self-care a priority by incorporating activities that nourish your body, mind, and spirit into your daily routine. This could include exercise, healthy eating, adequate sleep, relaxation techniques, or pampering yourself with a favorite activity.

Limit Exposure to Negative Influences: Be mindful of the media, social media, or toxic relationships that may contribute to negative emotions or stress. Set boundaries around your media consumption and choose to surround yourself with positivity whenever possible.

Seek Professional Support When Needed: If you're struggling to cope with difficult emotions or facing significant challenges, don't hesitate to seek support from a therapist, counselor, or mental health professional. They can provide guidance, validation, and coping strategies tailored to your specific needs.

Remember that emotional self-care is an ongoing process that requires attention and intentionality. By prioritizing your emotional well-being and practicing self-care regularly, you can cultivate greater resilience and thrive in all aspects of your life.

The Power of Positive Thinking: Positive thinking is a powerful mindset that can have profound effects on your mental and emotional well-being, as well as on your overall quality of life. Why positive thinking is important and how you can harness its power:

Enhanced Resilience: Positive thinking can boost resilience by helping you reframe challenges as opportunities for growth. Instead of seeing setbacks as insurmountable obstacles, a positive mindset allows you to approach them with optimism and determination.

Improved Mental Health: Cultivating a positive outlook can reduce symptoms of anxiety and depression, enhance self-esteem, and promote overall psychological well-being. By focusing on the good in your life and practicing gratitude, you can shift your perspective away from negative thoughts and emotions.

Better Physical Health: Research suggests that positive thinking can have tangible effects on physical health, such as strengthened immune function, reduced risk of cardiovascular disease, and increased longevity. A positive mindset is associated with healthier lifestyle choices, such as regular exercise, balanced nutrition, and adequate sleep.

Increased Happiness and Fulfillment: Positive thinking can lead to greater feelings of happiness, fulfillment, and life satisfaction. By focusing on the present moment and finding joy in everyday experiences, you can cultivate a sense of gratitude and contentment that enriches your life.

Improved Relationships: A positive attitude can enhance your relationships with others by fostering empathy, kindness, and cooperation. People are naturally drawn to those who radiate positivity, and maintaining a positive outlook can strengthen connections and build social support networks.

To harness the power of positive thinking in your life, consider incorporating the following practices:

Practice Gratitude: Take time each day to reflect on the things you're grateful for, whether it's the support of loved ones, moments of joy, or simple pleasures. Cultivating an attitude of gratitude can shift your focus away from negativity and foster feelings of abundance and appreciation.

Challenge Negative Thoughts: Become aware of negative thought patterns and challenge them with more balanced, realistic perspectives. Instead of dwelling on pessimistic or catastrophic thinking, look for evidence that contradicts your negative beliefs and focus on solutions rather than problems.

Cultivate Optimism: Cultivate a hopeful outlook by focusing on positive possibilities and reframing setbacks as temporary and surmountable. Practice visualizing success and envisioning positive outcomes for your goals and aspirations.

Surround Yourself with Positivity: Seek out uplifting influences, such as supportive friends, inspiring books, or motivational quotes.

Surrounding yourself with positivity can reinforce your own positive mindset and provide encouragement during difficult times.

Practice Self-Compassion: Treat yourself with kindness and understanding, especially when facing challenges or setbacks. Practice self-compassionate self-talk and offer yourself the same care and support you would give to a friend in need.

By cultivating a positive mindset and integrating these practices into your daily life, you can harness the transformative power of positive thinking to enhance your well-being, resilience, and overall quality of life.

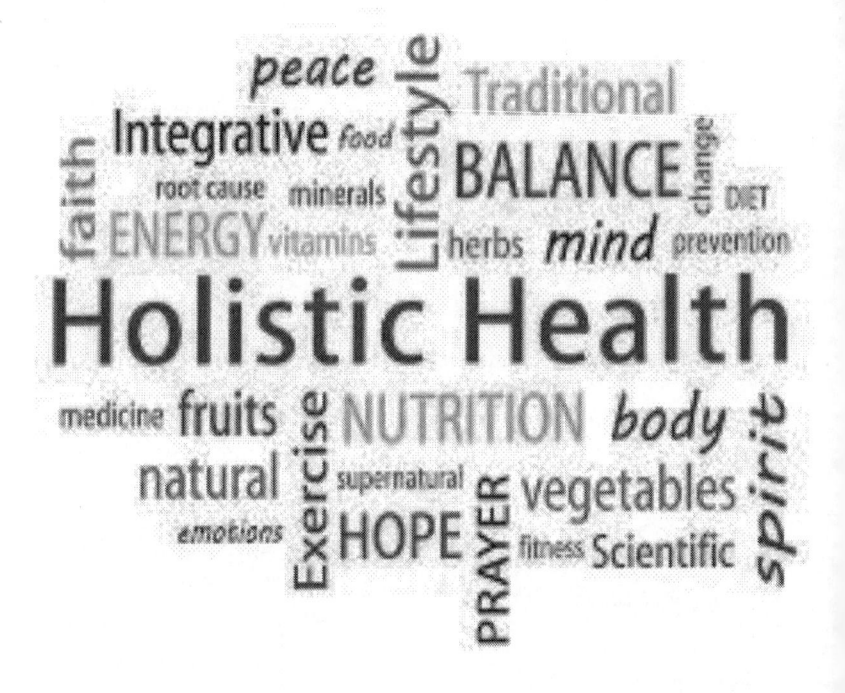

CHAPTER FOUR

Physical Vitality and Movement

Finding Joy in Movement: Finding joy in movement can be such a beautiful experience! Whether it's dancing, walking, swimming, or practicing yoga, movement offers a myriad of benefits beyond just physical health. Ways to find joy in movement:

Explore Different Activities: Try out various activities until you find the ones that resonate with you. Maybe it's a dance class, hiking in nature, or playing a sport with friends.

Focus on the Present Moment: Engage fully in the movement you're doing. Pay attention to how your body feels, the rhythm of your breath, and the sensations you experience. Being present can make the activity more enjoyable.

Set Realistic Goals: Set achievable goals that challenge you just enough to keep you motivated but are also realistic. Celebrate your progress along the way, no matter how small.

Find a Community: Joining a group or finding a workout buddy can add an element of social connection and accountability to your movement routine. Sharing experiences and cheering each other on can make the process more enjoyable.

Listen to Music: Create a playlist of your favorite songs or find music that energizes you and makes you want to move. Music can enhance your mood and make movement feel more like dancing.

Embrace Variety: Don't be afraid to mix things up and try new activities. Adding variety to your routine can prevent boredom and keep things exciting.

Practice Gratitude: Be grateful for your body's ability to move and all the sensations it allows you to experience. Cultivating gratitude can help you find joy in even the simplest movements.

Celebrate Your Achievements: Whether it's reaching a fitness milestone or simply making it through a challenging workout, take time to acknowledge and celebrate your achievements. Positive reinforcement can keep you motivated and make movement feel rewarding.

Connect with Nature: Take your movement outdoors whenever possible. Whether it's going for a run in the park or practicing yoga in your backyard, connecting with nature can enhance the experience and uplift your mood.

Listen to Your Body: Pay attention to how your body feels and honor its needs. Rest when you need to rest, and push yourself when you feel capable. Learning to listen to your body's cues can help you find joy in movement while also preventing injury.

Exploring Different Forms of Physical Activity: Exploring different forms of physical activity is a fantastic way to keep your fitness routine fresh, challenge your body in new ways, and discover what activities you truly enjoy. Forms of physical activity you might consider exploring:

Dance: Dancing is not only a great workout but also a fun way to express yourself. You can try various styles like salsa, hip-hop, ballet, or even Zumba.

Yoga: Yoga offers a combination of physical postures, breathing exercises, and meditation. It's excellent for improving flexibility, strength, and mental well-being.

There are many types of yoga, from gentle Hatha to vigorous Vinyasa.

Martial Arts: Martial arts like karate, taekwondo, or Brazilian jiu-jitsu not only provide a great workout but also teach discipline, focus, and self-defense skills.

Outdoor Activities: Explore outdoor activities such as hiking, biking, rock climbing, or kayaking. Not only do they provide physical benefits, but they also allow you to connect with nature.

Team Sports: Joining a recreational sports team can be a fun way to stay active while also fostering social connections. Consider sports like soccer, basketball, volleyball, or softball.

Strength Training: Incorporate strength training into your routine using bodyweight exercises, free weights, resistance bands, or weight machines. Building strength can improve overall fitness and help prevent injuries.

Pilates: Pilates centers on enhancing core strength, flexibility, and bodily consciousness. This low-impact exercise regimen is advantageous for individuals at any level of fitness.

Swimming: Swimming provides a comprehensive workout for the entire body while being gentle on the joints. Whether you're doing laps in the pool or trying water aerobics, swimming is a refreshing way to stay active.

Group Fitness Classes: Explore different group fitness classes offered at gyms or community centers. From spinning and kickboxing to circuit training and boot camps, there's something for everyone.

Mind-Body Practices: Besides yoga, explore other mind-body practices like Tai Chi or Qigong. These gentle movements can improve balance, coordination, and relaxation.

Remember to listen to your body and choose activities that you genuinely enjoy. Mixing and matching different forms of physical activity can keep your fitness routine exciting and sustainable in the long term.

The Benefits of Regular Exercise: Regular exercise offers a multitude of benefits for both your physical and mental well-being.

Improved Physical Health: Regular exercise helps to strengthen your heart, lungs, and muscles, improving cardiovascular health and reducing the risk of chronic diseases such as heart disease, stroke, type 2 diabetes, and certain cancers.

Weight Management: Engaging in physical activity helps to burn calories, control appetite, and maintain a healthy weight. When coupled with a well-rounded diet, consistent physical activity can aid in either shedding excess weight or sustaining a healthy weight.

Enhanced Mood: Exercise stimulates the release of endorphins, neurotransmitters in the brain that promote feelings of happiness and reduce stress and anxiety. It can also increase the production of serotonin and dopamine, which contribute to improved mood and mental well-being.

Better Sleep: Regular physical activity can improve the quality of your sleep by promoting relaxation and reducing insomnia. It helps regulate your sleep-wake cycle and enhances the overall duration and depth of sleep.

Increased Energy Levels: Engaging in regular exercise boosts your energy levels by improving circulation, delivering oxygen and nutrients to your tissues, and enhancing the efficiency of your cardiovascular system. It also increases your stamina and reduces fatigue.

Stronger Immune System: Moderate exercise has been shown to strengthen the immune system, making you less susceptible to infections and illnesses such as the common cold or flu. However, intense or prolonged exercise may temporarily suppress immune function, so it's essential to strike a balance.

Improved Cognitive Function: Exercise has cognitive benefits, including enhanced memory, concentration, and creativity. It promotes the growth of new brain cells and connections, particularly in areas associated with learning and memory.

Better Self-Esteem and Body Image: Regular physical activity can improve body image and self-esteem by helping you feel more confident and capable. Achieving fitness goals, gaining strength and flexibility, and seeing improvements in your physical appearance can boost self-confidence.

Social Connection: Participating in group fitness classes, sports teams, or outdoor activities provides opportunities for social interaction and can help build friendships and support networks. Social connection is essential for mental health and overall well-being.

Longer Life Span: Numerous studies have shown that regular exercise is associated with a reduced risk of premature death. Adopting a physically active lifestyle can increase your life expectancy and improve your quality of life as you age.

Incorporating regular exercise into your routine doesn't have to be complicated or time-consuming. Even small amounts of physical activity can provide significant health benefits. Aim for at least 150 minutes of moderate-intensity aerobic activity or 75 minutes of vigorous-intensity aerobic activity per week, along with muscle-strengthening activities on two or more days per week.

CHAPTER FIVE

Nurturing Relationships and Community

Nurturing relationships and fostering a sense of community are vital aspects of human well-being.

The Importance of Social Connections:

Emotional Well-being: Humans are social creatures, and meaningful connections with others fulfill your need for companionship, belonging, and intimacy. Strong social connections contribute to your overall emotional well-being, providing support during difficult times and enhancing your enjoyment of life.

Mental Health: Loneliness and social isolation are linked to a variety of mental health issues, including depression, anxiety, and low self-esteem. In contrast, having a network of supportive relationships can buffer against stress, improve mood, and promote psychological resilience.

Physical Health: Research has shown that social connection is associated with better physical health outcomes. People with strong social ties tend to have lower rates of chronic diseases, faster recovery times from illnesses, and longer lifespan. Social support can also encourage healthier behaviors, such as regular exercise and seeking medical care when needed.

Cognitive Function: Engaging in social activities and maintaining social relationships can help keep your brain sharp and may lower the risk of cognitive decline as you age. Social interaction stimulates mental processes, such as problem-solving, memory, and perspective-taking, which are important for cognitive health.

Quality of Life: Having meaningful relationships and a sense of community enriches your life in numerous ways. It provides opportunities for laughter, shared experiences, and personal growth. Feeling connected to others fosters a sense of purpose and fulfillment, enhancing your overall quality of life.

In summary, social connection is essential for your emotional, mental, and physical well-being. Prioritizing relationships and nurturing social ties can have profound benefits for your health and happiness.

Building Supportive Relationships:

Building supportive relationships is fundamental for personal well-being and resilience. Some key principles to consider:

Trust and Respect: Trust is the foundation of any supportive relationship. Establishing trust involves being reliable, honest, and respecting each other's boundaries and confidentiality.

Effective Communication: Open and honest communication is essential for building supportive relationships. Practice active listening, express yourself clearly and respectfully, and encourage the other person to do the same. Communication should be two-way, with both parties feeling heard and understood.

Empathy and Understanding: Empathy involves understanding and sharing the feelings of another person. Cultivate empathy by actively trying to see things from the other person's perspective, acknowledging their emotions, and providing validation and support.

Offering and Receiving Support: Supportive relationships involve both giving and receiving support. Be willing to offer assistance, encouragement, and a listening ear when needed, and don't hesitate to reach out for support yourself when you're facing challenges.

Boundaries: In healthy relationships, there's a mutual respect for each other's boundaries and autonomy. Establish clear boundaries and communicate them openly. Respect the boundaries of others and avoid pressuring them to disclose more than they're comfortable with or to take on more than they can handle.

Conflict Resolution: Conflicts are a natural part of any relationship, but they can be resolved constructively in supportive relationships. Approach conflicts with empathy, active listening, and a willingness to find mutually satisfactory solutions. Concentrate on understanding each other's viewpoint and seeking common ground.

Shared Values and Goals: Building supportive relationships is easier when there are shared values, interests, and goals.

Cultivate common interests and activities that bring you closer together and strengthen your connection.

Consistency and Commitment: Consistency and commitment are key to building and maintaining supportive relationships over time. Make an effort to stay in touch regularly, show up for each other, and prioritize the relationship despite life's challenges and busy schedules.

By prioritizing trust, communication, empathy, and mutual support, you can build strong, supportive relationships that enhance your well-being and resilience.

Communication Skills for Healthy Interactions: Communication skills are essential for fostering healthy interactions and relationships. Some key skills to focus on:

Active Listening: Actively listen to what the other person is saying without interrupting or forming your response while they speak. Give them your full attention, maintain eye contact, and use verbal and nonverbal cues to show that you're engaged and understanding.

Empathy: Try to understand the other person's viewpoint and emotions. Put yourself in their shoes and validate their feelings, even if you don't agree with them. Empathetic communication fosters trust, connection, and mutual respect.

Clarity and Conciseness: Express yourself clearly and directly, using simple and straightforward language. Steer clear of ambiguous statements that may cause confusion. Be clear and concise, sticking to the main point without unnecessary elaboration.

Nonverbal Communication: Pay attention to your body language, facial expressions, and tone of voice, as they can convey as much or more information than your words. Maintain open body language, such as facing the person, nodding, and smiling when appropriate, to show that you're engaged and approachable.

Respectful Feedback: Provide feedback in a constructive and respectful manner, focusing on behaviors or actions rather than criticizing the person's character. Employ "I" statements to communicate your thoughts and emotions without assigning blame or presuming intentions.

Assertiveness: Assertive communication involves expressing your thoughts, feelings, and needs in a confident and respectful manner while also respecting the rights and boundaries of others. Practice assertiveness by stating your opinions clearly, advocating for yourself, and setting boundaries when necessary.

Cultural Sensitivity: Be mindful of cultural differences in communication styles, norms, and expectations. Respect and accommodate cultural differences to ensure effective and respectful communication across diverse backgrounds.

Flexibility and Adaptability: Be flexible and adaptable in your communication style to meet the needs and preferences of different individuals and situations. Adjust your approach based on the context, relationship dynamics, and the other person's communication style.

By honing these communication skills, you can cultivate healthier and more fulfilling interactions with others, fostering stronger relationships and promoting mutual understanding and respect.

CHAPTER SIX

Environmental Harmony

Creating a Healthy Living Environment: Creating a healthy living environment involves several key aspects, encompassing both physical and mental well-being. Tips to help you create a healthy living space:

Cleanliness: Regularly clean your living space to remove dust, dirt, and other allergens that can affect air quality and contribute to respiratory issues.

Good Ventilation: Ensure proper ventilation in your home to circulate fresh air and prevent the buildup of indoor pollutants. Open windows when possible and use exhaust fans in areas like kitchens and bathrooms.

Natural Light: Maximize natural light exposure in your home, as it can positively impact mood and overall well-being. Consider using light-colored curtains or blinds that allow sunlight to filter through.

Indoor Plants: Incorporate indoor plants into your living space to improve air quality and reduce stress. Certain plants, like spider plants and peace lilies, are known for their air-purifying properties.

Reduce Toxins: Minimize exposure to harmful chemicals by choosing eco-friendly cleaning products, paints, and furnishings. Look for products labeled as non-toxic or low VOC (volatile organic compounds).

Healthy Eating: Stock your kitchen with nutritious foods and make it easy to prepare healthy meals. Keep fresh fruits and vegetables on hand and limit processed and high-sugar foods.

Regular Exercise: Create space for physical activity in your home, whether it's a designated workout area or simply enough room to stretch and move. Incorporate exercise into your daily routine to promote fitness and well-being.

Comfortable Sleep Environment: Invest in a comfortable mattress and pillows to ensure a restful night's sleep. Keep your bedroom dark, quiet, and at a comfortable temperature to promote quality sleep.

Stress Reduction: Create designated spaces for relaxation and stress relief, such as a cozy reading nook or a meditation corner. Incorporate calming elements like soft lighting, comfortable seating, and soothing decor.

Positive Relationships: Foster positive relationships with family, friends, and neighbors to create a supportive and nurturing environment. Spend quality time together and communicate openly to maintain strong connections.

Work-Life Balance: Establish boundaries between work and leisure time to prevent burnout and maintain overall well-being. Create a dedicated workspace if you work from home and prioritize activities that bring you joy and fulfillment.

Safety Measures: Ensure that your home is safe and secure by installing smoke detectors, carbon monoxide detectors, and security systems. Regularly check and maintain these devices to keep your living environment safe.

By incorporating these tips into your daily life, you can create a healthy living environment that promotes physical and mental well-being for you and your loved ones.

Connecting with Nature: Connecting with nature is essential for overall well-being and can be achieved in various ways, even if you live in an urban environment. Ideas to help you connect with nature:

Outdoor Activities: Spend time outdoors engaging in activities such as hiking, biking, jogging, or simply taking a leisurely walk in a park. Immersing yourself in natural surroundings can help reduce stress and improve mood.

Gardening: Start a garden, whether it's a small container garden on your balcony or a larger plot in your yard. Gardening allows you to connect with the earth, cultivate plants, and observe the wonders of nature up close.

Nature Walks: Take regular nature walks to explore nearby trails, forests, or botanical gardens. Pay attention to the sights, sounds, and smells of the natural world around you, and take time to appreciate its beauty.

Birdwatching: Set up a bird feeder or bird bath in your yard or balcony to attract birds. Spend time observing and identifying different bird species, and keep a journal of your sightings.

Outdoor Yoga or Meditation: Practice yoga or meditation outdoors to combine the benefits of mindfulness with the calming effects of nature. Find a quiet spot in a park or garden where you can practice in tranquility.

Beach Trips: If you live near the coast, take advantage of beach trips to relax by the water, listen to the sound of waves, and soak up the sun. Swimming, beachcombing, and building sandcastles are activities that can help you feel connected to the natural world.

Nature Photography: Bring a camera or Smartphone with you on outdoor excursions to capture images of landscapes, plants, animals, and other natural elements. Photography can deepen your appreciation for the beauty of nature and provide a creative outlet.

Stargazing: Spend evenings stargazing in an area with minimal light pollution. Use a telescope or binoculars to observe celestial objects such as stars, planets, and constellations, and marvel at the vastness of the universe.

Nature Retreats: Consider going on a nature retreat or camping trip to immerse yourself fully in the natural environment. Disconnect from technology and embrace the simplicity of life outdoors.

Environmental Conservation: Get involved in environmental conservation efforts in your community, such as volunteering for park cleanups or participating in tree planting initiatives. Taking action to protect and preserve nature can foster a deeper sense of connection and stewardship.

Regardless of where you live or how much time you have, finding ways to connect with nature can have profound benefits for your physical, mental, and emotional well-being. Prioritize spending time outdoors and nurturing your connection with the natural world.

Sustainable Living Practices: Sustainable living practices are essential for reducing your environmental footprint and preserving natural resources for future generations. Sustainable living practices you can incorporate into your daily life:

Reduce, Reuse, Recycle: Follow the three Rs of waste management by reducing consumption, reusing items whenever possible, and recycling materials such as paper, glass, plastic, and metal.

Conserve Energy: Reduce energy consumption by turning off lights, appliances, and electronics when not in use. Replace traditional incandescent light bulbs with energy-efficient LED or CFL bulbs, and consider installing programmable thermostats to optimize heating and cooling.

Water Conservation: Conserve water by fixing leaks, taking shorter showers, and installing water-saving devices such as low-flow faucets, showerheads, and toilets. Collect rainwater for gardening and landscaping purposes.

Eat Sustainably: Choose locally grown, organic, and seasonal foods whenever possible to support sustainable agriculture practices and reduce greenhouse gas emissions associated with food transportation. Decrease meat intake and integrate additional plant-based meals into your diet.

Compost: Compost organic waste such as fruit and vegetable scraps, coffee grounds, and yard trimmings to create nutrient-rich soil for gardening. Composting diverts waste from landfills and reduces methane emissions.

Use Eco-Friendly Transportation: Walk, bike, carpool, or use public transportation to reduce reliance on fossil fuel-powered vehicles. Consider investing in electric or hybrid vehicles if feasible, and combine errands to minimize driving.

Choose Sustainable Products: Purchase products made from renewable materials, recycled content, or biodegradable materials. Look for eco-friendly certifications such as Energy Star, Forest Stewardship Council (FSC), and USDA Organic.

Reduce Single-Use Plastics: Minimize the use of single-use plastics such as plastic bags, bottles, and packaging. Opt for reusable alternatives such as cloth bags, stainless steel water bottles, and glass containers.

Support Sustainable Fashion: Choose clothing made from sustainable and ethical materials such as organic cotton, hemp, bamboo, or recycled fibers. Buy fewer items of higher quality and donate or recycle clothing you no longer need.

Conscious Consumerism: Practice mindful consumption by considering the environmental and social impact of your purchases. Support companies and brands that prioritize sustainability, fair labor practices, and ethical production methods.

Green Your Home: Make your home more energy-efficient by improving insulation, sealing air leaks, and installing energy-efficient windows and appliances. Consider investing in renewable energy sources such as solar panels or wind turbines.

Educate Yourself and Others: Stay informed about environmental issues and share your knowledge with friends, family, and community members. Encourage others to adopt sustainable living practices and advocate for policies that promote environmental conservation.

CHAPTER SEVEN

Integrating Holistic Wellness into Daily Life

Practical Tips for Everyday Holistic Living: Holistic living is about nurturing your mind, body, and spirit in harmony with the natural world. Some practical tips for incorporating holistic practices into your everyday life:

Mindfulness Meditation: Take a few minutes each day to practice mindfulness meditation. Focus on your breath and observe your thoughts without judgment. This can help reduce stress and increase self-awareness.

Nutritious Diet: Eat whole, unprocessed foods such as fruits, vegetables, whole grains, and lean proteins. Avoid excessive consumption of processed foods, sugars, and artificial additives. Stay hydrated by drinking plenty of water throughout the day.

Regular Exercise: Engage in physical activity that you enjoy, whether it's yoga, walking, swimming, or dancing. Exercise not only strengthens your body but also boosts your mood and improves mental clarity.

Quality Sleep: Prioritize sleep by establishing a regular sleep schedule and creating a relaxing bedtime routine. Aim for 7-9 hours of quality sleep each night to support overall well-being.

Stress Management: Practice stress-reduction techniques such as deep breathing exercises, yoga, tai chi, or progressive muscle relaxation. Find activities that help you unwind and manage stress effectively.

Creative Expression: Explore your creative side through activities such as painting, writing, music, or crafting. Creative expression can be therapeutic and nourish your soul.

Limit Screen Time: Reduce the amount of time spent on electronic devices, especially before bedtime. Instead, engage in activities that promote relaxation and mental stimulation, such as reading a book or practicing a hobby.

Remember that holistic living is about finding balance and harmony in all aspects of your life. Start small and gradually incorporate these practices into your daily routine to experience the benefits over time.

Overcoming Common Obstacles: Overcoming obstacles is a natural part of life, and when it comes to embracing holistic living, there can be specific challenges. Some common obstacles and tips for overcoming them:

Time Constraints: Many people struggle to find time for self-care and holistic practices amidst busy schedules. To overcome this obstacle, prioritize your well-being by scheduling time for activities like meditation, exercise, and healthy meal preparation. Even dedicating just a few minutes each day can make a difference.

Financial Constraints: Holistic living can sometimes involve expenses such as gym memberships, organic foods, or wellness classes. Look for affordable alternatives such as free community events, online resources, or DIY home practices. Additionally, focus on simple, budget-friendly habits like walking in nature, practicing gratitude, and cooking at home.

Lack of Motivation: It's common to feel unmotivated at times, especially when starting new habits or overcoming challenges. Break down tasks into smaller, achievable steps and acknowledge your progress as you go. Find inspiration from others who share similar goals, and remind yourself of the benefits you'll experience by prioritizing your well-being.

Social Pressure: Peer pressure or societal norms may discourage holistic practices or healthy choices. Surround yourself with supportive individuals who respect your lifestyle choices, and gently educate others about the benefits of holistic living if they express skepticism. Remember that your well-being is ultimately your priority, regardless of others' opinions.

Overwhelm: The vast amount of information available on holistic living can sometimes feel overwhelming. Start with one or two practices that resonate with you and gradually incorporate more over time. Focus on what feels manageable and sustainable for your lifestyle, and don't hesitate to seek guidance from trusted sources or professionals if needed.

Self-Doubt: Doubts or negative self-talk can sabotage your efforts to embrace holistic living. Practice self-compassion and cultivate a positive mindset by acknowledging your strengths and progress.

Surround yourself with affirmations, supportive communities, or mentors who uplift and encourage you on your journey.

Old Habits: Breaking old habits and establishing new ones can be challenging. Be patient with yourself and understand that change takes time. Identify triggers that lead to unhealthy habits and develop strategies to replace them with healthier alternatives. Stay committed to your goals, and celebrates each small victory along the way.

By recognizing and addressing these common obstacles, you can overcome barriers to holistic living and create a more balanced and fulfilling lifestyle. Remember that every step forward, no matter how small, brings you closer to your well-being goals.

Creating a Personalized Wellness Plan: Creating a personalized wellness plan involves identifying your individual needs, goals, and preferences, and then developing strategies to support your overall well-being. Step-by-step guide to help you create a personalized wellness plan:

Assess Your Current State: Take stock of your current lifestyle, including your physical health, mental well-being, stress levels, sleep quality, diet, exercise habits, and social connections. Reflect on what areas of your life could use improvement and what aspects you're already satisfied with.

Set Specific Goals: Based on your assessment, identify specific and measurable goals that you want to achieve in various areas of your life. For example, your goals might include improving your fitness level, reducing stress, getting better sleep, or adopting healthier eating habits. Make sure your goals are realistic and achievable within a reasonable timeframe.

Identify Your Priorities: Determine which aspects of your well-being are most important to you and prioritize them accordingly.

You may choose to focus on one area at a time or work on multiple goals simultaneously, depending on your capacity and preferences.

Develop Action Steps: Break down each of your goals into smaller, actionable steps that you can take to move closer to achieving them. Ensure that these actions are Specific, Measurable, Attainable, Relevant, and Time-bound (SMART). For example, if your goal is to improve your fitness level, your action steps might include scheduling regular exercise sessions, joining a gym or fitness class, and tracking your progress.

Explore Holistic Practices: Consider incorporating a variety of holistic practices into your wellness plan to address different aspects of your well-being. This might include mindfulness meditation, yoga, tai chi, aromatherapy, massage therapy, acupuncture, journaling, or spending time in nature. Experiment with different practices to see what resonates with you and what brings you the most benefit.

Create a Routine: Establish a daily or weekly routine that includes your chosen wellness practices and activities. Schedule time for self-care and prioritize your well-being just like you would any other important commitment. Consistency is key to seeing results and maintaining positive habits over the long term.

Track Your Progress: Keep track of your progress toward your goals by regularly monitoring your actions and outcomes. This could involve keeping a journal, using a wellness app or tracker, or simply checking in with yourself regularly to reflect on how you're doing. Celebrate your successes along the way and adjust your plan as needed based on your evolving needs and circumstances.

Seek Support: Don't hesitate to reach out for support from friends, family members, or professionals who can help you stay accountable and provide encouragement along your wellness journey. Consider joining a support group, hiring a coach or therapist, or participating in workshops or classes related to your goals.

Be Flexible and Adapt: Life is unpredictable, and it's normal to encounter setbacks or challenges along the way. Be flexible and willing to adapt your wellness plan as needed to accommodate changes in your circumstances or priorities. Remember that progress is not always linear, and it's okay to adjust your goals and strategies as you learn and grow.

Practice Self-Compassion: Be kind to yourself throughout this process and recognize that wellness is a journey, not a destination. Embrace imperfection and give yourself grace when things don't go as planned. Celebrate your efforts and achievements, no matter how small, and remember that every step forward counts toward improving your overall well-being.

By following these steps and tailoring them to your unique needs and preferences, you can create a personalized wellness plan that supports your holistic well-being and helps you live a healthier, happier life.

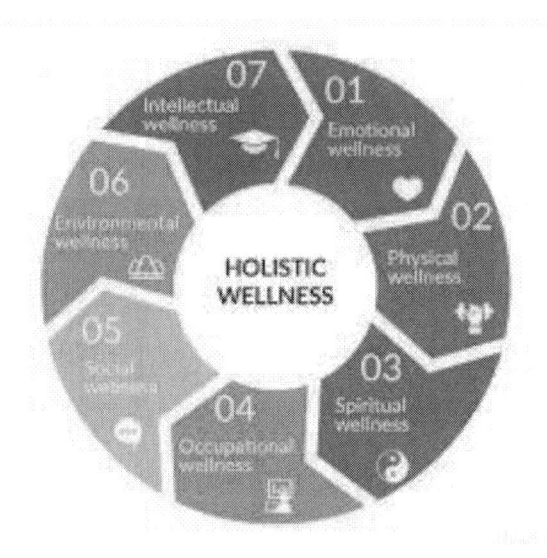

CHAPTER EIGHT

Beyond the Self: Holistic Wellness for the Greater Good

The Ripple Effect of Your Wellness: The ripple effect of your wellness refers to the idea that when you prioritize your own well-being and take steps to improve your physical, mental, and emotional health, it can have positive effects that extend beyond you and influence others around you, as well as larger communities.

Here's how the ripple effect of your wellness works:

Personal Well-Being: When you focus on your own wellness, you often experience improvements in various aspects of your life, such as increased energy, better mood, higher productivity, and reduced stress.

Positive Influence: As you become healthier and happier, you naturally radiate positive energy and inspire those around you. Others may be motivated to adopt similar healthy habits or seek support to improve their own well-being.

Relationships: Wellness practices can strengthen interpersonal relationships. For example, someone who prioritizes self-care may have more patience, empathy, and resilience in their interactions with others, leading to healthier and more fulfilling relationships.

Workplace Environment: In a professional setting, employees who prioritize wellness are often more engaged, focused, and collaborative. Their positive attitude and productivity can create a more supportive and vibrant workplace culture, inspiring colleagues to also prioritize self-care.

Community Impact: As more individuals prioritize wellness, it can contribute to the overall health and vitality of communities. Healthy and engaged individuals are more likely to participate in community activities, support local initiatives, and contribute positively to the social fabric.

Long-Term Benefits: The ripple effect of your wellness can have long-lasting effects on society as a whole. By promoting healthier lifestyles and positive behaviors, it can lead to reduced healthcare costs, lower rates of chronic diseases, and a more resilient and thriving population.

Ultimately, the ripple effect of your wellness highlights the interconnectedness of your experiences and the powerful influence that personal choices can have on the well-being of oneself and others. By nurturing your own wellness, you can create a ripple effect of positivity and inspiration that extends far beyond your immediate circles.

Advocacy and Activism for a Healthier World: Advocacy and activism for a healthier world involve individuals and groups taking action to promote policies, practices, and behaviors that contribute to improved health and well-being on a global scale. Here are some key aspects of advocacy and activism in this context:

Awareness Campaigns: Advocates and activists often initiate awareness campaigns to educate the public about health issues, such as the importance of physical activity, nutritious eating, mental health awareness, and access to healthcare services. These campaigns aim to raise awareness, reduce stigma, and mobilize support for positive change.

Policy Advocacy: Advocates work to influence policies at local, national, and international levels to address systemic factors that impact health, such as poverty, inequality, environmental pollution, and inadequate healthcare infrastructure. This may involve lobbying policymakers, mobilizing public support, and participating in legislative processes to advocate for evidence-based policies that promote health equity and social justice.

Community Empowerment: Activists often focus on empowering communities to take control of their health by providing resources, education, and support for grassroots initiatives. This may include organizing community health fairs, supporting local farmers' markets, advocating for safe recreational spaces, and promoting access to affordable healthcare services.

Social media and Digital Activism: In today's interconnected world, social media and digital platforms play a crucial role in advocacy and activism for a healthier world. Activists use these platforms to raise awareness, share information, mobilize support, and amplify voices that might otherwise be marginalized.

Hashtags, online petitions, and viral campaigns can help generate momentum and spark meaningful conversations about health-related issues.

Intersectionality and Inclusivity: Effective advocacy and activism recognize the intersectionality of health issues and prioritize inclusivity and diversity. This means considering how factors such as race, ethnicity, gender, sexual orientation, disability, and socioeconomic status intersect to influence health outcomes. Advocates strive to address systemic inequalities and ensure that health interventions are accessible and culturally appropriate for all individuals and communities.

Global Collaboration: Many health challenges, such as infectious diseases, climate change, and access to essential medicines, require global cooperation and collaboration. Advocates and activists work across borders to share knowledge, resources, and best practices, advocate for international treaties and agreements, and hold governments and corporations accountable for their actions that impact global health.

Overall, advocacy and activism for a healthier world involve a multifaceted approach that encompasses raising awareness, influencing policies, empowering communities, leveraging digital platforms, promoting inclusivity, and fostering global collaboration. By working together, individuals and groups can contribute to creating a more equitable, sustainable, and healthier future for everyone.

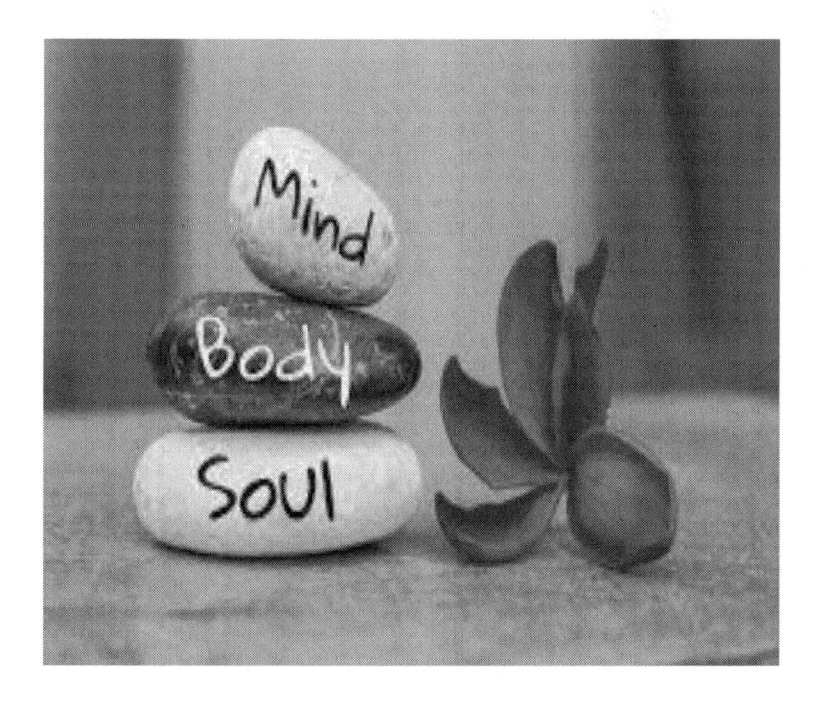

CONCLUSION

Embracing Wholeness

Reflecting on Your Journey to Holistic Wellness: Reflecting on my journey to holistic wellness is a deep move into understanding the interconnectedness of my physical, mental, emotional, and spiritual well-being. It's about recognizing that each facet of my being influences the others and striving for balance and harmony in all aspects of my life.

Physically, I've learned the importance of nourishing my body with wholesome foods, staying active, and getting enough rest. I've come to appreciate the intricate relationship between nutrition, exercise, and sleep in maintaining optimal health.

Mentally, I've explored various practices like meditation, mindfulness, and cognitive-behavioral techniques to cultivate a positive mindset and manage stress. Developing resilience and the ability to adapt to life's challenges has been key in my journey toward mental wellness.

Emotionally, I've embraced the full spectrum of human emotions, allowing myself to feel and express them in healthy ways. I've learned to practice self-compassion, acceptance, and forgiveness, both toward myself and others, fostering emotional resilience and well-being.

Spiritually, I've transformed into practices that nourish my soul and connect me to something greater than myself. Whether through meditation, prayer, or spending time in nature, I've found solace and meaning in cultivating a deeper spiritual connection.

Overall, my journey to holistic wellness has been a transformative experience, guiding me toward a more balanced and fulfilling life. It's an ongoing process of self-discovery, growth, and self-care, where each day presents new opportunities to nurture and nourish all aspects of my being.

Committing to Ongoing Growth and Self-Discovery:
Committing to ongoing growth and self-discovery is a pledge to embrace the journey of becoming the best version of oneself. It involves a mindset of continuous learning,

exploration, and evolution, acknowledging that personal growth is a lifelong process.

One aspect of this commitment is to remain open to new experiences and perspectives. It means stepping out of comfort zones, trying new things, and being willing to learn from successes as well as failures. Every experience, whether positive or negative, offers an opportunity for growth and self-discovery.

Self-reflection is another vital component. Taking the time to introspect, evaluate values, beliefs, and behaviors, allows for deeper understanding of oneself and fosters personal growth. It's about asking tough questions, confronting limitations, and striving for self-improvement.

Setting goals and striving for progress is integral to ongoing growth. Whether small or ambitious, goals provide direction and motivation, driving continual development. Celebrating achievements along the way reinforces commitment and encourages further growth.

Additionally, seeking inspiration and guidance from mentors, role models, and resources can fuel personal development. Learning from others' experiences, wisdom, and expertise can broaden perspectives and accelerate growth.

Lastly, embracing resilience and adaptability is crucial in the journey of ongoing growth. Life is full of twists and turns, and being able to navigate challenges with resilience and flexibility enables one to continue progressing despite setbacks.

Committing to ongoing growth and self-discovery is not always easy, but it is immensely rewarding. It leads to greater self-awareness, fulfillment, and a deeper sense of purpose in life. As long as one remains dedicated to the journey, the possibilities for growth are endless.

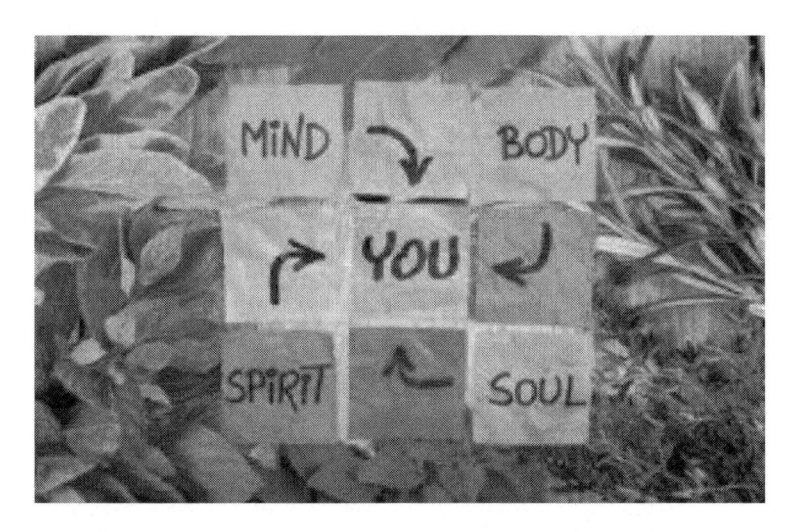

Printed in Great Britain
by Amazon